YOGA

WITH YOUR

CAT

YOGA WITH YOUR CAT

Text by Elanor Clarke

Illustrations by Tetiana Svirska

An Hachette UK Company
www.hachette.co.uk

Summersdale Publishers Ltd
Part of Octopus Publishing Group Limited
Carmelite House
50 Victoria Embankment
LONDON
EC4Y 0DZ
UK

www.summersdale.com

Printed and bound in China

ISBN: 978-1-78783-645-7

Substantial discounts on bulk quantities of Summersdale books are available to corporations, professional associations and other organizations. For details contact general enquiries: telephone: +44 (0) 1243 771107 or email: enquiries@summersdale.com.

YOGA
WITH YOUR
CAT

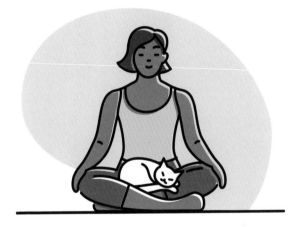

SAM HART

Illustrations by Tetiana Svirska

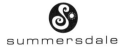

summersdale

INTRODUCTION

We all know that cats are devotees of the deep stretch and masters of mischief, so this book combines two of their favourite things! You might actively choose to involve your kitty in your yoga practice, or they might just have a sixth sense for when it's time to interfere. Whatever your situation, the simple guidance and gorgeous illustrations in this book will show you just some of the ways that cats and yoga can mix. Read on for tips on how to achieve the perfect pose (or asana) from both the hatha and vinyasa traditions of yoga.

Please remember, before you start a new form of exercise, to check with your doctor, particularly if you have a pre-existing health condition. Correct form, including hand placement, must be used, and practitioners should only attempt poses they feel comfortable with — never force yourself into a pose, particularly an advanced one. Breathing is just as important to yoga as the movements and holds, so focus on your breathing, keeping it deep and even. Most of all, though, enjoy the sense of focus, balance and relaxation you can achieve with yoga, even if your cat insists on "helping"!

CHILD'S POSE
Balasana

The child's pose is a very relaxing position, which provides a degree of relief to counter some of the strong bends in yoga — it can also be a great place to start a yoga practice,' as it brings you to stillness and presence. It gently stretches and lengthens the spine, hips and ankles, and can help to relieve back pain, which many of us suffer with. Balasana also allows us to reconnect and ground ourselves. Watch out for your kitty companion, though — your outstretched hands may look perfect for pouncing on!

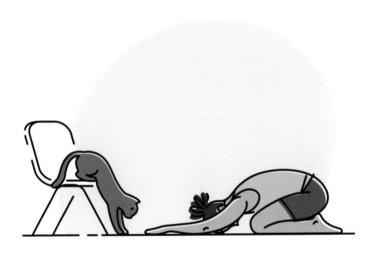

STAFF POSE
Dandasana

Dandasana is the basis for many seated yoga poses, helping your body to maintain good seated posture. Sitting with legs outstretched and using the arms for support, you lengthen and strengthen the spine. This simple yet effective position also allows you to open the chest and exercise your stomach muscles. Be careful about how long you sit in this pose, as your feline friend might see it as a good opportunity to test your poise — *let me see, where can I balance?*

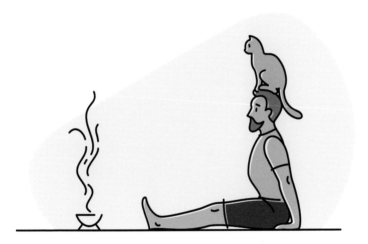

RAISED ARMS POSE

Hasta Uttanasana

Forming a core part of the sun salutation series often used in hatha yoga, hasta uttanasana is a full-body stretch and gentle backbend. It helps warm up the body for more intense poses, opens up the chest, allowing for deeper breathing, and helps strengthen the spine, improving posture. Cats much prefer it when you're bending forwards to stroke their heads — they may be confused about why you would be choosing to lean away from them when they are right there.

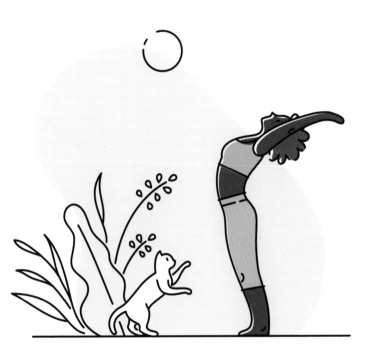

DOWNWARD-FACING DOG

Adho Mukha Svanasana

One of the key poses within the sun salutation sequence, and an integral part of most practitioners' mat time, downward-facing dog is a simple yet challenging pose, which offers full-body stretching and toning. As well as stretching the entire length of the spine, it strengthens the arms and legs. To avoid pressure on the shoulders imagine a string pulling your hips skywards. Needless to say, your kitty will be unimpressed. Dog? No, no, no.

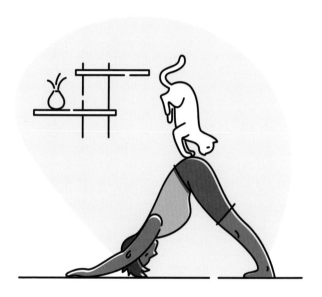

CAT POSE
Marjaryasana

This book simply wouldn't be complete without the feline's firm favourite. Cat pose is usually paired with cow pose, and the gentle movement between the opposing back stretches helps increase the spine's flexibility, as well as warming up the body. In marjaryasana, on all fours, we curve the spine upwards, like a cat mid-stretch. Of course, your furry companion is going to want to join you for this one — after all, we learned it from them!

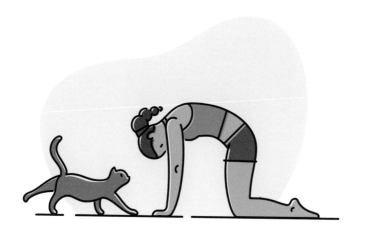

COW POSE

Bitilasana

A strange pairing in the animal kingdom, but the counter to cat pose is cow pose. Allow the spine to bend downwards, and open the chest up and out, before rhythmically stretching back into cat pose. Not only does your spine get a lovely gentle release, but the exercise allows for deep and relaxed breathing, and meditative focus. Cats are going to wonder why you don't stick to cat pose, though — they can vouch for it being the best stretch.

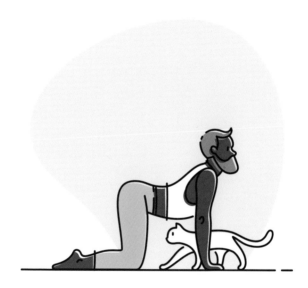

COBRA POSE

Bhujangasana

A very deep back stretch, cobra lengthens and tones lots of areas: obviously the back (expect a release of lower-back tension), but also the buttocks and shoulders. It helps open up the chest, allowing you to breathe deeper, and is believed to help with digestion by stimulating the abdominal organs. Feline friends love this pose and will inevitably want to help out.

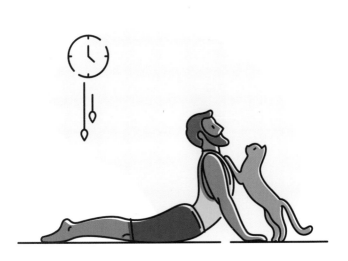

SPHINX POSE

Salamba Bhujangasana

Similar to cobra, but with more support and a less extreme backbend, sphinx pose is great for beginners who wish to start lengthening their spine and improving its flexibility. It also opens the chest and shoulders, and it's very aptly named, as you can see. Why not try it with your own little furry sphinx? The regal pose comes so easily to them...

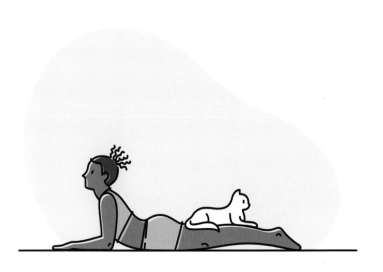

HALF LORD OF
THE FISHES POSE

Ardha Matsyendrasana

A slightly simpler version of Lord of the Fishes pose, this seated twist is named after a master yogi from around the tenth century. It stretches the hips, spine, shoulders and neck, is believed to help relieve fatigue, and is recommended for menstrual cramps, as it squeezes and engages the abdomen. It is an ideal pose to counter the aches and pains of day-to-day life, particularly for those who sit at a desk all day. Added benefit: your flat knee makes an ideal chin rest for your cat companion.

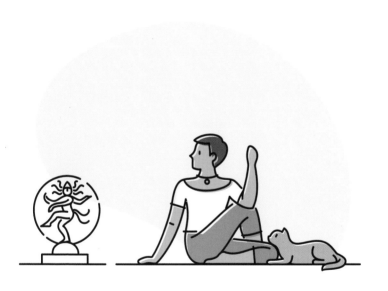

BRIDGE POSE
Setu Bandha Sarvangasana

A great backbend for beginners which fits well within any yoga practice, bridge is a beneficial posture than has also found its way into other forms of exercise as a way to stretch and strengthen the back, legs and backside. It also works on the abdominal muscles and can relieve neck tension. The pose can be made more challenging by a kitty settling on your raised abs — let's face it, all surfaces are cat beds.

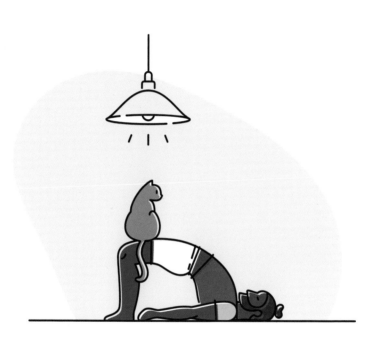

25

TREE POSE
Vriksasana

Tree pose is a simple single-foot balance which is suitable for beginners. It strengthens the standing leg and ankle, builds up awareness (you may lose balance if your mind wanders) and, of course, helps improve equilibrium. Many find this position meditative. Your kitty, though, might just wonder why you're standing so still and not playing with them — leg climbing is not unheard of!

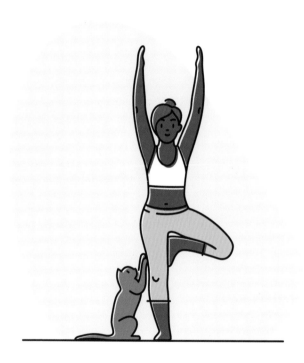

FOUR-LIMBED STAFF POSE

Chaturanga Dandasana

Part of the sun salutation, chaturanga dandasana is akin to a low plank. It is important to use good form, otherwise this pose can result in shoulder injuries. Done correctly, though, chaturanga has a host of strength benefits, particularly for the shoulders, arms, wrists, core and lower back. It also strengthens the muscles around the spine, and so can help improve posture. You're creating such a nice flat surface with your back in this position; don't be too surprised if you become an impromptu cat bed!

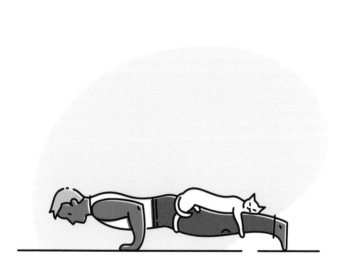

BOW POSE

Dhanurasana

Thus named because your body resembles a bow ready to be fired in this position, bow pose is an excellent backbend. These are particularly beneficial as, unlike forward bends, we are unlikely to move our bodies in this way in day-to-day life, so they're a great way to counter rounded shoulders and back pain associated with, for example, computer work. Dhanurasana stretches the entire front of the body and encourages flexibility in the spine. Your cat's probably bemusedly wondering why your legs are in the air, but you aren't on your back — *humans are weird.*

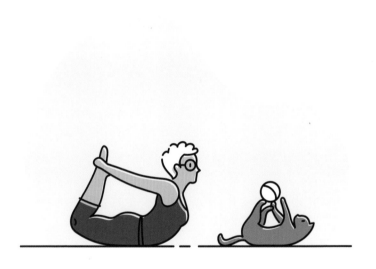

SEATED
FORWARD BEND
Paschimottanasana

A deep bend, which stretches the back, legs and shoulders, seated forward bend is a simple concept that can take a long time to master. It is important to never force your body fully into the position; as long as your form is good and you are feeling the stretch, you will begin reaping the benefits. This pose is believed to alleviate stress, and can help with menstrual cramps by stimulating the area in question. Unfortunately, you're likely to look like a handy springboard for your cat, so don't be too surprised if they leap up.

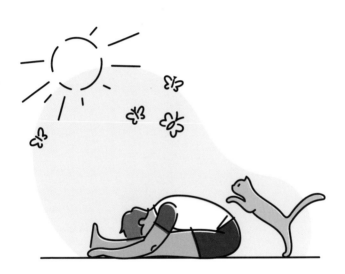

EQUESTRIAN POSE

Ashwa Sanchalanasana

A deep lunge, the equestrian pose is another in the sun salutation sequence of hatha yoga. It improves the spinal musculature (which can even make you stand taller), improves back flexibility, opens out the hips, and strengthens the knees and ankles. It also promotes core strength and opens out the chest to allow deeper breathing. While you are so close to the ground, your kitty might be thinking that it's playtime — *why aren't you pouncing, human?!*

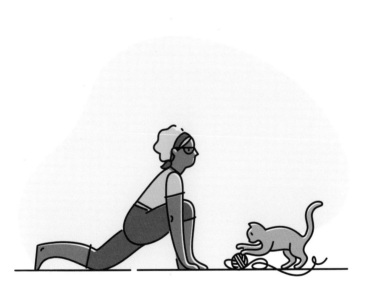

LOCUST POSE
Salabhasana

An excellent backbend to help less experienced yogis prepare for more intense poses such as the wheel (page 88), locust pose helps improve strength and flexibility in the entire back side of the body, including the legs, buttocks and back, thus leading to better posture. Your cat will look wholly unimpressed by this pose — don't worry, it's just because they know you've exceeded their ability on this occasion; there's no way they could achieve this.

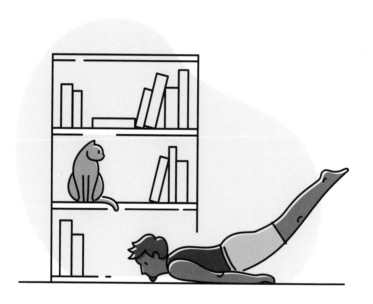

STANDING HALF FORWARD BEND
Ardha Uttanasana

Like most forward bends, ardha uttanasana stretches and lengthens the legs — including those areas, such as the hamstrings, which get particularly tight from sitting all day in desk jobs. It also stretches the front of your torso, and your lower back, really helping release tension in those problem areas while building strength. Not to mention, it's the ideal position for gazing lovingly at kittens — what more could you need?

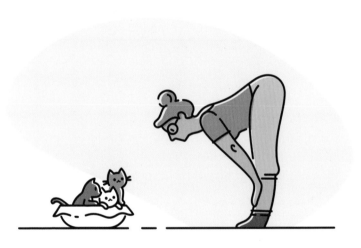

EXTENDED PUPPY POSE

Uttana Shishosana

An excellent position for beginners, or just to add a gentle spinal stretch to your practice, extended puppy pose is a wonderful combination of downward-facing dog (page 12) and child's pose (page 6). It opens the shoulders, improves flexibility and deepens relaxation. Even though you'll look a lot like a luxuriating cat, if your feline friends catch wind of the name this one's going on the banned list, too. Kitten poses only!

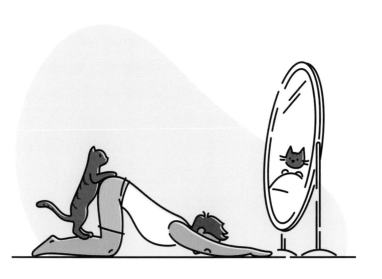

WARRIOR I POSE

Virabhadrasana I

There are three warrior poses — in this first pose, your arms reach towards the sky, like the warrior's raised sword. Being a lunging position, warrior I strengthens the legs in particular, but also opens up the hips and chest. It is a great position for developing a feeling of groundedness, and it helps improve balance. Plus, your low, lunged position makes a perfect cat hiding place, somewhere to lurk before they pounce!

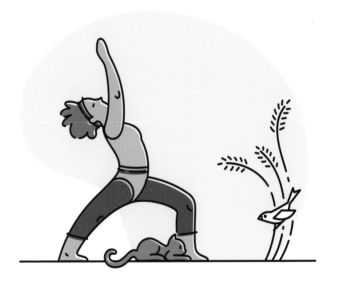

WARRIOR II POSE
Virabhadrasana II

In this second of the three warrior poses, we are metaphorically pulling back an arrow to fire it. The position helps improve balance, strengthens the legs and shoulders, and opens out the chest. It also deeply stretches the groin — an area where tension is held and we often end up pulling muscles when we start exercising. Why not up the difficulty by being weighted? Cats make excellent shoulder weights.

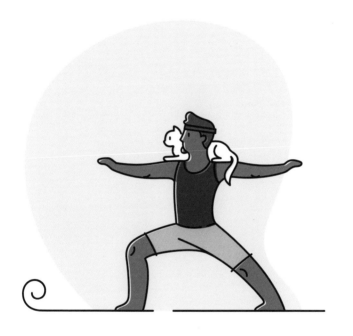

WARRIOR III POSE
Virabhadrasana III

In the last of the three warrior poses, you are the embodiment of the arrow in flight. It works the whole body, incorporating strength and balance. Warrior III encourages better posture, coordination between different parts of the body, improved balance and increased endurance. Warning: you may look like a cat tree and fall victim to some clawed climbing during this pose!

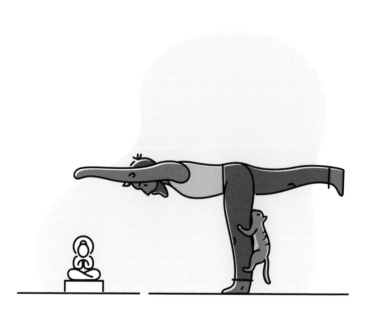

REVOLVED HAND-TO-BIG-TOE POSE

Parivrtta Hasta Padangusthasana

A single-foot balance, this pose helps improve leg and core strength, flexibility in the hips (among other areas) and awareness of the position and movement of the body. It also works the glutes hard, helping develop a strong backside — which is great for easing lower-back pain. If you can't fully stretch and reach your toes, it can be adapted by keeping the leg bent and holding the knee. Plus, with that outstretched hand you can always multitask with a favourite cat dangler...

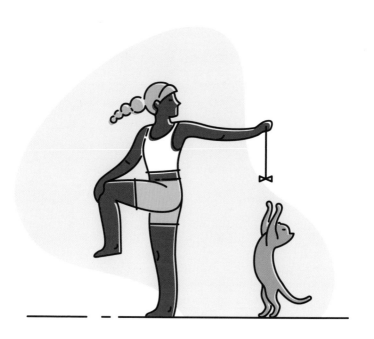

SUPPORTED SHOULDER STAND

Salamba Sarvangasana

The shoulder stand is one of the key inverted yoga positions. Inversions (turning your body upside down) help improve circulation, balance and relaxation. It is believed a shoulder stand can also relieve a headache, so it's a great addition to your evening practice after a hard day's work. In this version you use a blanket for support, reducing the pressure through your shoulders and neck. Best to be sure your feline friend is not sitting under you when you release this position — neither of you would appreciate the results!

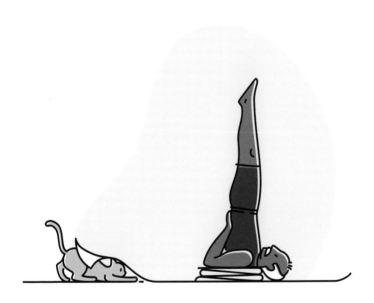

REVERSE
TABLE TOP
Ardha Purvottanasana

A great way to balance out all those forward bends in your yoga practice, reverse table top also engages the core and strengthens the wrists and the legs, while also energizing you. It is a fantastic pose for those of us who sit at a computer all day, as it combats the shoulder slump and rounding of the back we may experience, helping us stand tall. Pro tip: if you have long hair, a bun is ideal for this pose — your kitty companion may see that ponytail as a great new toy to catch...

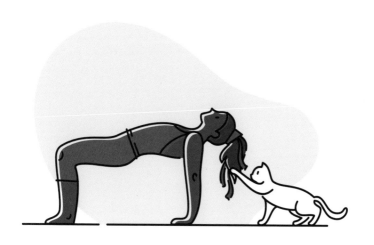

CHAIR POSE
Utkatasana

Often referred to as „fierce„ pose from the Sanskrit *utkata*, meaning „powerful„ or „difficult„, this standing position challenges the legs in particular. It works the hip flexors, thighs and gluteals to strengthen and stabilize the pelvis, an area where we commonly store stress. Don't expect any feline sympathy while you work; the likeliest scenario is this: you pose as the chair, they'll sit on a nearby perch and gloat.

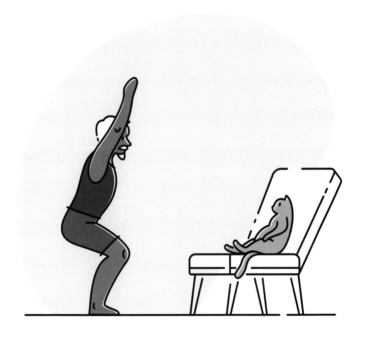

GATE POSE

Parighāsana

Gate pose is a side stretch, which opens out the whole side of the torso from your hips right through to your fingertips. A shoulder opener, it also helps alleviate neck tension. If you find this uncomfortable on the kneeling knee, you could always place a blanket under it for additional support. Watch out, though — that exposed armpit could be a prime spot for unexpected tickles from nosy kitty whiskers!

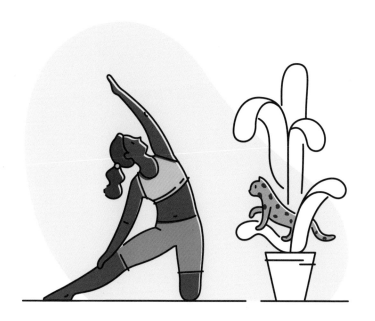

NOOSE POSE

Pasasana

In this position, you may genuinely feel that you've tied your body in a knot! This twisting posture deeply stretches the upper body, and needs a firm foundation, with your feet planted on the ground. The twist may remind you of how cats manage to scratch everywhere with that one back foot and make it seem so effortless!

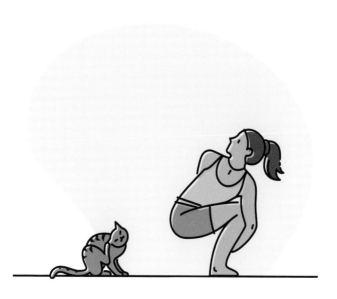

LORD OF THE DANCE POSE
Natarajasana

Sometimes referred to as dancer pose, this position combines a backbend with a balance, and can be challenging for beginners. Natarajasana brings a host of benefits — not only does it improve balance and focus, it also strengthens the legs, opens the chest and helps improve back flexibility. Make sure your foot is planted directly beneath your hips to achieve this pose. Your kitty knows they look so much more graceful than you doing this, but cats are like liquid — we just can't compete...

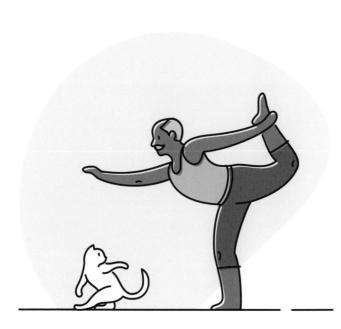

SHOULDER STAND

Sarvangasana

Like the supported shoulder stand earlier in this book, the full shoulder stand is an inversion, with all the benefits associated with turning your body upside down, such as increased flow of blood to the brain, improvement in circulation and strengthening of the back. Cats may wonder why they're looking at your feet instead of your face — an upside-down human is very confusing.

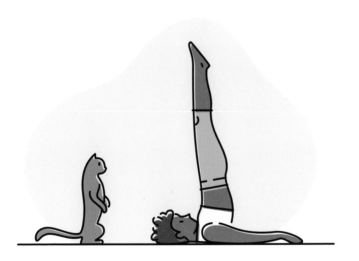

PEACOCK POSE
Mayurasana

An advanced two-handed balance suitable only for experienced yogis, peacock pose particularly challenges and strengthens the wrists, arms and shoulders. It is also great for the core, and stimulates the digestive organs, so is believed to aid digestion and reduce constipation. Watch out for hidden kitties when releasing this position — they may be soft, but we don't want to squash them!

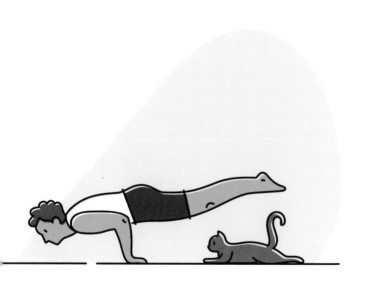

REVOLVED
TRIANGLE POSE

Parivrtta Trikonasana

This position has a host of benefits, as it combines twisting, bending and stretching to work multiple muscle groups and allow deep opening of the hips, shoulders and chest. Opening the chest encourages deeper breathing and is a great counterbalance for modern life, where we often sit hunched, closing our chest and not taking in as much oxygen. This position is also believed to stimulate the abdominal organs, helping the digestion process — an all-round health boost. The likelihood is, though, your cat is just going to wonder what you're pointing at and be disappointed it isn't a bird.

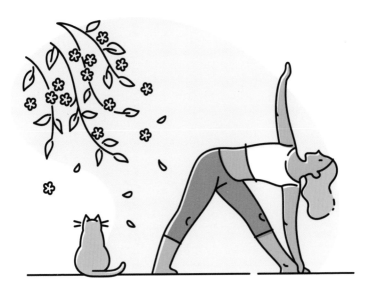

SUPPORTED HEADSTAND

Salamba Sirsasana

For some, the headstand is the ultimate inverted position and, as such, should never be attempted by a novice — indeed some never achieve a headstand, but still gain the benefits of less intense inversions. Headstands can be hard on your neck, and must be practised safely with expert guidance — preferably with a tutor. If done right, they are highly beneficial and relaxing. They increase blood flow to the head, are believed to help relieve stress, and improve digestion, as well as strengthening the shoulders, neck, back and abdominals. Watch out for kitty projectiles, though — that's one way to lose your focus!

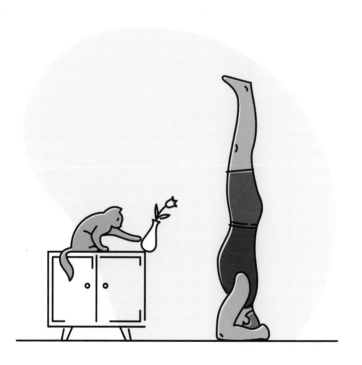

CORPSE POSE
Savasana

Though it may look unbelievably simple, corpse has often been described as the most difficult yoga poşe. While there is no contortion or balancing involved in lying flat on your mat, the goal of savasana is to observe good posture while engaging in complete relaxation. For many yoga students, relaxing both body and mind is one of the most challenging things you can do. Having cats in the house probably only makes it harder — you know they just love to *boop!* a sleepy face.

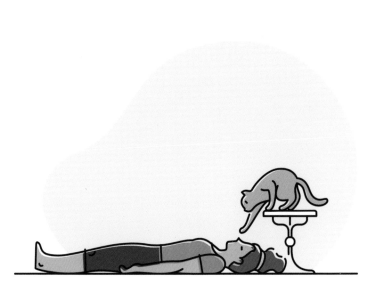

PLANK POSE
Phalakasana

The plank is a superstar yoga position, with an incredible array of benefits. Not only is it one of the best exercises for improving core strength, in practising it you will also gain better balance and improve posture. The added benefit of lengthening the spine in this position is reduced back pain. Beware, though, your cat might see you as the perfect climbing opportunity — weighted plank, anyone?

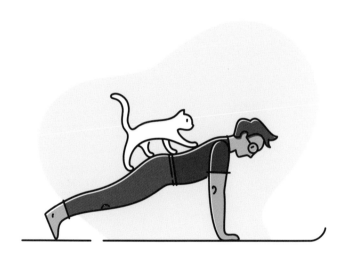

FISH POSE

Matsyasana

Often used as a counter to the shoulder stand, which can put a strain on the shoulders, fish pose stretches and releases them. It encourages flexibility in the upper spine and shoulders, and even stretches the intercostals (the muscles between the ribs). Lying on the floor with the back arched upwards, this position resembles a fish, but we all know this is not the kind of fish your cat is after...

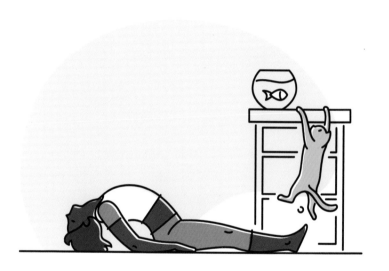

BOAT POSE

Navasana

An intense position for your abdominal muscles in particular, boat pose is one of the more challenging yoga positions, but offers a real sense of satisfaction when it can be held. It also strengthens the spine and hips, as the mid-body must work effectively together to maintain the strength and balance needed to hold this position. Your cat is unlikely to "help"; they'll probably just wonder what on earth you're doing, while being sure that, if they tried, they could definitely do it better.

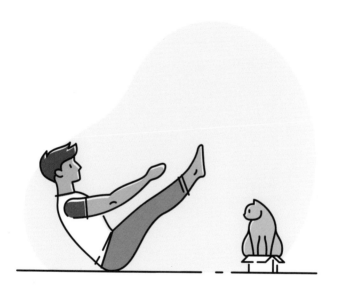

HERON POSE
Krounchasana

Heron pose offers deep stretches to strengthen multiple areas. In the extended leg, the hamstrings and gluteals are the main focus (a block can be used under the backside to help with the extension), while the bent leg works the quads. The position also strengthens the muscles in the lumbar region of your back, where most of us bipeds experience back pain. Felines rejoice! The humans finally got the memo on how best to bathe. Just look at that leg!

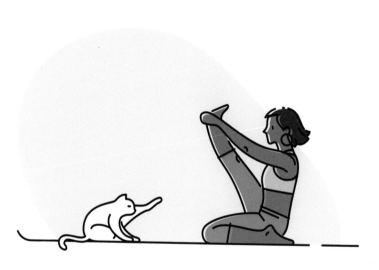

SCORPION POSE
Vrschikasana

This is a very challenging pose, and definitely for advanced practitioners only, combining elements of backbends and inversions and requiring incredible strength and focus — eventually, practitioners are able to touch their feet to their heads in this position. If you're able to perform it, vrschikasana provides a deep stretch through most of the body, helping to build balance, flexibility and strength, including in the core and lower back. Watch out for cats trying to "help" you get your feet just that little bit closer to your head!

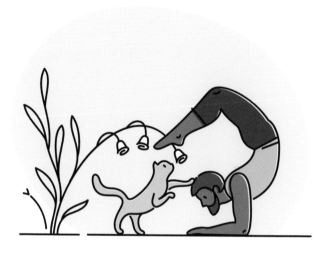

REVOLVED
HALF-MOON POSE
Parivrtta Ardha Chandrasana

A challenging, deeply strengthening combination of balance, rotation and stretch, this is a position which offers full-body toning and flexibility. If you have difficulty reaching the floor with your hand, you can adapt this position by using a block to ease the downward stretch. Try not to let snuffling whiskers tickle your foot — it might make it harder to hold your balance!

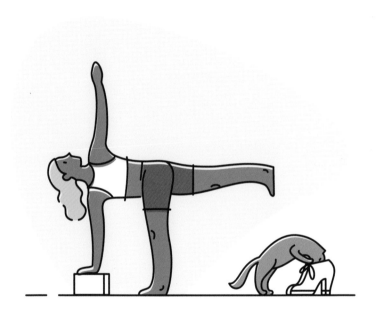

PLOUGH POSE

Halasana

Though it may look difficult, the plough pose is very relaxing — it stretches the spine and shoulders, reducing tension and easing nerves. Often used towards the end of daily practice, it helps get you ready for deep relaxation. Relaxation may be hard to attain, though, if your raised backside looks like a handy perch for your kitty — watch out for those claws!

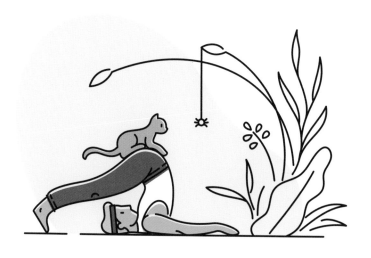

CAMEL POSE

Ustrasana

This is an energizing position which stretches the entire front of the body and increases flexibility in the spine. It is another pose believed to help improve digestion. Furthermore, it's a great counter to the multiple forward bends that most yoga practices entail. All cats know the benefits of a nice long back stretch — this one definitely goes on the approved list.

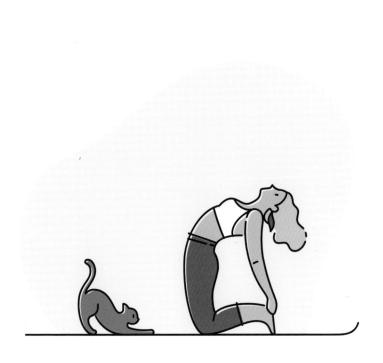

WHEEL POSE
Urdhva Dhanurasana

A strong, invigorating backbend, the wheel (or "upward bow") is usually the first pose in the ashtanga vinyasa yoga sequence — a modern-day form of traditional Indian yoga. However, it's a more advanced pose and beginners may find this challenging. Urdhva dhanurasana opens the chest, stretches and lengthens the back, and strongly works the shoulder muscles. It can also help relieve lower-back pain. This is one cats understand well — turning upside down is second nature for them.

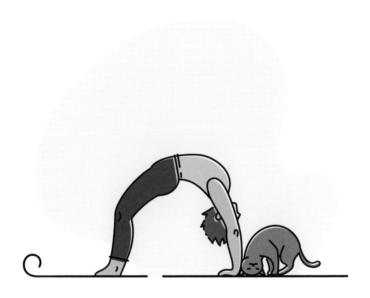

MONKEY POSE
Hanumanasana

Named for the monkey god Hanuman and based on his mythological "leap of faith", monkey pose is a challenging asana which opens out the hips into a split. This should never be forced, and it's best to adapt the pose to suit your own level of flexibility, gradually working on softening your joints. This pose also deeply stretches the hamstrings, which are often very tight for most of us. Be warned, though, with limbs everywhere, you're going to become an ideal climbing frame for kittens!

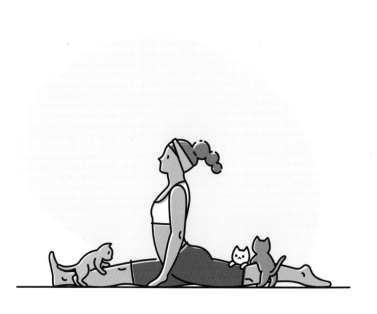

CROW POSE

Bakasana

Crow pose is a daring and challenging double-hand balance. The name is actually derived from the Sanskrit for crane, as the pose is believed to resemble a crane wading through the water. This asana strengthens the arms, tones the abdominal muscles and opens the groin. It helps develop your sense of balance, and it builds focus. Warning: may scare cats — you suddenly look like a giant frog that could leap on them at any moment!

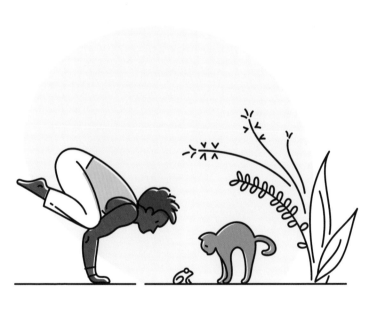

EASY POSE
Sukhasana

Sometimes called "the pose of happiness", sukhasana is a simple, comfortable cross-legged seated position used for grounding, relaxing and connecting. As well as being used at the beginning of most yoga practices, it is a position often employed to complete your practice. Using your palms to rub and warm your legs and arms, place them over your eyes and breathe in the warmth, then sit in meditation — namaste. And as we all know, a pair of crossed legs makes the perfect little nest for a sleeping cat... Bliss.

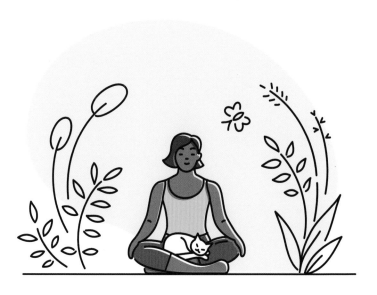

If you're interested in finding out more about our books, find us on Facebook at **Summersdale Publishers** and follow us on Twitter at **@Summersdale**.

www.summersdale.com

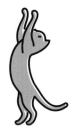